The Ultimate Skin Picking Cure Guide

I0439786

How to Overcome Compulsive Picking and Dermatillomania for Life

Table of Contents

Introduction

The pages in this short, concise book are intended to help people who want to better understand how a compulsive skin picker thinks, how skin picking becomes an addiction, as well as strategies to overcome these issues.

Compulsive skin picking is not as heavily researched by scientists as many other addictions or disorders, and some people who don't have to deal with the problem blow it off, because it does not seem very serious from an outside perspective.

People who suffer from compulsive skin picking have a tendency to hide the disorder from friends, family members, and even their doctors. As a result, there is not much information regarding ways to treat it directly. But the available treatments target the need to change habits and manage emotions in order to stop the compulsion behind skin picking.

You will find this book useful if you make sure to implement what you learn in the following pages. Compulsive skin picking is not conquered overnight, but the important thing to remember is, it is definitely possible for you to overcome it. The information presented in this book is for you to better understand your own mind and body, as well as the steps you will need to make your journey.

As you go through these pages, you'll get a better understanding of what skin picking really is and where it stems from, as well as learn several ways that you can begin to overcome it. We will dive into what is going on in your brain, how your body reacts to your triggers, how your childhood can influence you, as well as what work is required of you to get past the roadblocks you have.

It is recommended that you take notes while reading the book. This will ensure that you get the most out of the information in here. The notes will help you to pinpoint exactly what you need to implement and by writing things down, you will be able to recall specifics and how to handle certain situations when they arise.

Lastly, it is encouraged that you do your own research into the topics that you want to look deeper into. The more you understand your own mind and body, the better off you'll be. To overcome compulsive skin picking, it will take some work on your part, but you can do it! So remember to read with confidence and an open mind!

Chapter 1:

What Is Compulsive Skin Picking?

Skin picking is a disorder that is characterized by the constant fussing over, scratching, digging into, rubbing, and poking of one's skin to the point of damage. It is also known as dermatillomania, excoriation, neurotic excoriation, and compulsive skin picking (CSP), acne excoriee, pathological skin picking (PSP), and psychogenic excoriation.

The primary target of a skin picker is the face, but as it is a disorder, other parts of the body that contain skin are also targeted.

People with a skin picking disorder pick on existing elements on the skin, like moles and freckles, or fledgling skin conditions, such as acne, skin sores and scabs, using their hands, particularly the fingernails. Some people use their teeth or devices like tweezers, nail cutters, pins, needles, and other things to pick as well.

This results in contusions, discolorations, infections, scars, and other deformities of the skin. A certain area of the body can become covered with these deformities to the point where the person that is picking can feel quite self-conscious about his/her body.

The reason many people struggle to get help with this problem is because the more they engage in picking at their skin, the worse their skin gets, and the more self-conscious they become. This becomes a vicious cycle, and it usually doesn't end until the person suffering becomes fed up enough to finally take action and ask for help.

Before the skin picking occurs, the person experiences an extreme sense of compulsion or itchiness. During the course of skin picking, the person ultimately experiences a feeling of satisfaction and pleasure. A compulsive skin picking disorder is related to more serious psychological problems like depression, but it is a habit that is unconsciously triggered by a degree of tension and urge.

After the relief and satisfaction that skin picking brings to the individual, there typically comes a feeling of shame and self-consciousness, given the fact that the results are very tangible and apparent on the skin. During the act, the feeling of pleasure is too much for the person to stop, even if they know the feeling of shame will ensue.

People with a compulsive skin picking disorder may go to great lengths to hide their scars by putting on additional clothing or adding make-up to their faces, in order to cover the scars that their skin picking has left. However, this is just for the "normal", more common cases.

Unfortunately, sometimes a skin picking disorder can become a much larger problem. When skin picking gets worse, people often become anti-social, avoiding the presence of other people in situations where their skin marks may be seen, which could force them to uncomfortably explain their situation.

A person with a skin picking disorder has the capacity to damage his or herself and do it in a repetitive manner until the level of urge or compulsion is satisfied. It may seem like common sense from the outside looking in, but it is important to remember that when the urge comes to a picker, they are oftentimes unaware of their urges, until their skin begins to show noticeable signs on the outside.

In 1898, the French Dermatologist M.L. Brocq was believed to be the first one to describe the onset and effects of skin picking, also known as dermatillomania or excoriation disorder. He observed that some young and feeble girls who already had skin lesions actually worsened the said lesions by scratching and picking on them repeatedly.

He also observed that the people who were prone to doing this were also quite sensitive and repressive. Since they could not express themselves by means of conversing with others or being angry, they tended to release their built up stress on their own skin. When told not to, they often became hostile and vindictive. Oftentimes, they were also temperamental and moody, and tended to push others away just so they could be by themselves and pick their skin with no one watching.

It is said that the inability to control the urge to pick one's skin could be likened to hair pulling (trichotillomania). Early studies showed that apart from helping someone release their stress, skin picking may also be connected to heightening one's arousal.

The similarities stem from the fact that they're both "ritualistic", but without any obvious preceding obsessions, and that these compulsive actions are triggered the same way (i.e., by anger, loneliness, the need for self-destruction, etc). The main difference, though, is that skin picking is mostly suffered by females, whereas other compulsive behaviors are quite evenly spread throughout genders.

Some even liken it to Obsessive Compulsive Disorders, but the main difference, according to most experts, is that 1) OCD is never pleasurable while skin picking could be, 2) Those with skin picking disorder may prove to be harder to treat than those with OCD because they don't feel like something is really wrong with them, 3) Skin picking isn't usually driven by obsession, and 4) Skin picking may lead to addiction. This means that it may be caused by several psychological factors.

While picking the skin, the afflicted person may feel like he/she is in a trance because they get to be oblivious of whatever's going on around him/her, and only focuses on picking skin. Some even go to the lengths of harming or mutilating their own skin just so scabs would be formed and so they could pick the said scabs.

It is classified as one of the varieties of Body-Focused Repetitive Behaviors (BFRBs), which includes nail biting, hair pulling (trichotillomania), and biting the interiors of the cheeks. It is also important to know, this disorder can be triggered by feelings such as excitement, boredom, and anxiety, but it can also be an effect of a much more serious psychological problem.

This disorder is especially harmful to teenagers and young adults because it is done in a repetitive manner and for such a long time. This results, not only in obvious scars on the skin, but also in subsequent damage to a person's psychological health, as well as their social life. Research has shown that it can create tension and conflicts within a person's circle of interaction in their work environment, as well as in their school and family relationships.

A compulsive skin picking disorder is, indeed, a symptom of a more serious problem. It is still related to the aforementioned skin problems that are considered "more serious", but it can also be autoimmune related. Research has found that some people with substance abuse issues also pick their skin, as well as those with body dysmorphic disorder.

Needless to say, because of the diversity of its connections, it is important to identify where the problem of skin picking is related, as a symptom in order to identify the proper treatment. In other words, the best way to overcome a compulsive skin picking disorder is to identify where the issue is stemming from within the individual.

Diagnosis for skin picking is deemed complicated by many, because there are certain factors that need to be taken into consideration before saying that a person already has a skin picking disorder. This may include a doctor checking to see if a person has other underlying conditions, such as psoriasis, eczema, diabetes,

Hodgkin's Disease, Liver Disease, Systemic Lupus, Polycetemia Vera, and Prader-Will Syndrome.

More often than not, skin picking sufferers also pick on just one certain patch of the skin at a given time, filling it up with scabs and the like. Doctors would then check whether a person has been excessively picking on their face, lips, body, legs, or arms.

Examples of skin picking can be seen in the film *Black Swan*, where it is shown as a precursor of Nina's anxiety. It also became the subject of a couple episodes of *Obsessed*, a show that deals with the treatment of several anxiety disorders.

Chapter 2:

Causes of Skin Picking and How It Happens

To begin to understand the causes of skin picking, we must first realize it is important to understand a little bit about human psychology. The triggers that we all have as people are mostly noticeable by our outward expression to the world. In other words, we can usually tell that someone is lacking in confidence if they are slumped over all the time, even if we don't know much else about them.

Another example would be someone who looks away when they are talking to you. We understand that this usually means this person is either lacking in confidence (shy), or being deceitful. Now that we have a few examples of human psychology being expressed outwardly, let's focus on the causes of compulsive skin picking and how it tends to be expressed.

As mentioned earlier, skin picking begins for many reasons. For a lot of patients, it begins with the prevalence of acne. Due to the fact that acne is considered embarrassing by many, one begins to pick and scratch at his/her acne and thus, the compulsion begins. It becomes a defense mechanism against the acne as well as whatever people might say about it. People who pick their skin might feel like they are at least able to have some control over their situation.

Sometimes, skin picking develops because of other underlying conditions, such as psoriasis, keratosis, and eczema. Of course, when the said conditions are prevalent, one cannot deny the fact that the skin really needs to be groomed or picked.

The problem begins when the patient can no longer determine when he/she is helping themselves, versus when they are just picking skin out of habit. Again, one has to realize that this mostly stems during adolescence. At that point in one's life, a person is quite sensitive, especially when it comes to physical appearance.

Another cause of skin picking is that it is often a coping mechanism against stress or arousal or any other turmoil that one is facing at a certain moment in time. This then shows that the person has an impaired stress response, which is evident in picking the skin, which then causes tissue damage in the long run. Still, the afflicted person often denies that this is happening.

Some neurologists and psychologists also believe that skin picking may be caused by repressed rage toward authoritative figures in one's life. For example, when one has overbearing parents who pressure them to achieve, it can begin a cycle of suppression and repression.

If a youth knows that he/she can not live up to parents' expectations, that person may begin to build a shell or a wall around themselves and stays in that shell, picking skin in the process because he/she feels like it's one of the only things they can control.

OCD is also a big cause, since at least 53% of people who suffer from skin picking also suffer from OCD. But again, one must take note that they are two different things, although they could overlap in some cases.

Some studies show that those who have no cognitive flexibility differences but have less motor-inhibitory control are prone to develop skin picking compulsion. This has something to do with thinking about two different concepts in life. When one has less motor-control, it's obvious that it would be difficult for him/her to control themselves, especially when it comes to suppressing inappropriate behaviors.

Studies also show that there is a link between picking and dopamine. Dopamine is an organic chemical in the brain that has important roles in one's body. It is a neurotransmitter, which means that it has a lot to do with motor control and reward-motivated behavior.

When one is taking drugs, whether certain pharmaceutical ones, or prohibited ones such as methamphetamine or cocaine, can lead to uncontrollable picking, and may even lead to an extremely heightened sex drive. That said, a dysfunction towards dopamine functions may be largely at play when it comes to knowing whether a person can be afflicted with skin picking disorder or not.

There are also certain case studies showing that disabled people tend to pick their skin as a form of regaining control over their body. Since they believe their bodies have been disabled or harmed without them being able to do anything about it, they might feel like picking their skin is the only method they have of regaining control.

Body Dysmorphic Disorder is also said to be one of the potential causes of skin picking. The disorder essentially entails a person having a skewed perception of his/her own body. The perception doesn't have any basis in reality and could remain the same, despite a person making dramatic changes to their physique.

A person who suffers from BDD may often check themselves in the mirror to see what bad they could say about themselves, and are often fond of touching their skin to feel like they're real and to tell themselves that there's something they need to change about their body.

Too often, they also go into social withdrawal, because they feel like every person they meet has something bad to say about them - even if it couldn't be farther from the truth. Around 73% of people with this disorder tend to be more concerned with their skin than anything else - and are also prone to committing suicide.

When a person is anxious, tensed or stressed, he/she usually resorts to actions brought about by compulsion. This is common in all people, and we can find examples everywhere. Some people gamble, some play video games, and some bite their nails when they are anxious, tensed, or stressed. These are all examples of compulsive activities.

If you are suffering from a compulsive skin picking disorder, you may be taking out your anxieties, worries, or fears on your body instead of making an outward expression like maybe lifting heavy weights at the gym or running a mile. There may be two people with the same exact stressors in their lives, but they both may take it out differently. If you take out your stress in a way that can benefit you and the people around you, instead of a self-harming way, then you have won the battle. The problem is that most people are never able to replace that habit of picking with something more productive.

When a person gets the urge or the itch to scratch their skin, it is usually on a spot that already has a skin condition. Because the picking is done constantly and for a long period of time, the skin defect or condition that can otherwise heal on its own, will usually worsen by excessive bleeding or leaving marks and scars.

The more the person picks on that tender area, because of compulsion, the more the skin condition gets irritated and infected. And because the compulsion will not stop until it is satisfied on a psychological or emotional level, the skin condition will definitely progress for the worse, turning into skin defects and leaving noticeable marks on the skin in undesirable locations, like the arms, face, or legs.

People with this disorder typically have a favorite place on their skin to pick. However, because they leave so many marks on this common place, they often proceed to exploring some other part of their body. The result of this exploration is a massive sea of scars, begging to heal before they go through another round of picking.

Common recurring picking locations include the lips, arms, back, shoulders, stomach, legs, fingernails and toe nails, gums, and others.

Some people compulsively pick their skin in a certain area briefly, but repeatedly spread out the locations on their body during the day. Others will do it as little as one time in a day, but will pick in a certain area for hours on end with the use of fingernails or a favorite mechanical device like tweezers, needles, or pins.

Too much skin picking can worsen skin conditions, damaging the tissues involved. It may also lead to complications, such as septicemia, which is when the area of the body can become extremely inflamed because of an intense infection. When a person picks the skin for a long period of time, it can also result in epidural abscesses and skin grafting.

These extreme cases range from easily treatable to life-threatening situations, which can hospitalize a person if not treated quickly. This may sound scary to you, but remember that if you are suffering from compulsive skin picking, you have the chance to make a change before further damage is done. It is important to know the possible consequences so that you can avoid getting to these points.

Because the activity is done unconsciously most of the time, a person with a skin picking disorder is not usually aware of the consequences brought about by his/her skin picking, until it gets noticeably bad. Some cases have even been recorded where skin picking damages the neck and back muscles because of the sustained amount of effort and stress that a person exerts in order to satisfy their itch. They may stay in an uncomfortable position for minutes or hours on end, which can cause their body to develop muscular imbalances over time.

When a person feels guilty, ashamed, powerless, and humiliated, this can likewise trigger him/her to become even more compulsive in his/her actions, adding to the possibility of even more self-harm. Research has even shown that among people with dermatillomania, 12% entertain the idea of suicide, 11% of those try to commit suicide, while 15% undergo psychiatric treatment.

People with a compulsive skin picking disorder often feel guilty or ashamed after the activity or perhaps after seeing the damage it has brought to their skin. A common scenario of skin picking, not only leaves marks and infections on the person's skin, but also a lot of discarded skin on the floor. There are also people with this disorder that eat the skin, contributing further to the emotional turmoil of such activity.

Chapter 3:

Who Suffers From Compulsive Skin Picking?

Estimates of the general population that suffer from dermatillomania vary between different scientific institutions. However, in one study, it has been estimated that up to one in twenty people suffer from this addiction.

According to studies, this is most common among female adolescents, and could start as early as 10 years of age, and could be extremely prevalent between the ages of 15 to 20. It does not matter whether a person is physically healthy or not, as long as there are emotional or mental problems that leads him/her to skin-pick.

Upon comparing all studies, it is relatively fair to say that this disorder affects around 1.4 to 5% of the general population in the United States alone. Surveys showed that at least 16% of people afflicted with skin picking tend to pick their skin until they see noticeable tissue damage, because simply seeing blood alone is not enough for them. It is not just about hurting themselves, but mostly about being able to do what they want with their skin - again, it's about the feeling of "control".

For some people, it really starts with the onset of acne - but the behavior just does not go away even when they enter adulthood. Stressful events may also lead people from continuing to pick their skin, especially when it is something life-changing, such as: marriage, annulment, divorce, violence, or death. It should also be noted that in some rare cases, skin picking may be hereditary.

It can strike during childhood and throughout adulthood for any person. Nobody is really exempt from it, so if you are an older man, you shouldn't feel embarrassed that you are in the minority, as there are many other older men in the exact same situation as you. People often think that this only affects teenagers and young adults going through puberty, which simply isn't true.

People, generally, pick a specific location to scratch if that part of the skin already has a skin problem, such as a pimple or a rash. There is nothing wrong with this act, since many times, this is how a person would deal with having a new blemish like a pimple. However, it becomes a disorder when it causes damage, not just to the skin, but also in other areas of a person's life.

The skin, therefore, is not the sole problem. A compulsive skin picking disorder goes beyond a skin itch that if scratched goes away. Because the disorder is rooted from a more psychological level, it becomes a compulsive habit that's hard to break, even with the obvious scars that it has left all over a person's body. This is important to remember going forward.

When people with this disorder are asked about the experience, most of them say that skin picking is soothing and pleasurable. This pleasure satisfaction is experienced away from the mirror or any semblance of reflection, because the results and damage to such compulsive activity is very much apparent on the person's body.

Pickers become so enchanted in these extended moments, it becomes difficult to stop the pleasure. It can almost be related to an orgasm in the mind, which can become addicting after experienced enough.

While they are causing lesions, marks and infections on the skin, they are more focused on experiencing the trance that skin picking brings. It is, indeed, a pathological disorder that begins like a grooming habit that has gone to the extreme, and the compulsion that it brings results in feelings of guilt, shame, damaged self-esteem, and more damaging psychological problems within that person.

Studies continually try to classify compulsive skin picking disorder, primarily, because it is with the right classification that the right treatments can be identified. And although it is commonly classified under obsessive-compulsive disorders, new studies have shown that its symptoms exhibit neurobiological similarities to people with addictions. It is a disorder on its own, while also a disorder that can develop into other more serious disorders.

However, because of the shame and guilt that people feel after skin-picking, most people with this disorder deliberately fail to seek treatment, especially during the early stages of the sickness. And in medicine, if low cases are being disclosed, it is hard to conduct studies that can, consequently, lead to more treatments and cures.

Even worse, people with the disorder are usually unable to find others who can relate to the same situation, because they are too ashamed to tell another person in the first place. It is a cycle of withdrawal that prevents anyone from the outside to be able to relate with the picker.

As it continually becomes more difficult to treat this disorder through new medications, researchers use antidepressants and cognitive-behavioral therapy in their studies to find the most effective treatments.

Chapter 4:

Skin Picking as a Symptom to Other Disorders

Obsessive Compulsive Disorder

People that have a compulsive skin picking disorder find pleasure and satisfaction from an activity that is, obviously, painful and disturbing. The truth is, the act of harming yourself and still being comfortable and emotionally fulfilled by doing so is truly abnormal.

It is hard to avoid the compulsion, let alone stop it. This is the reason the person continues to wallow in the pain, even as the feelings of guilt and shame set in.

The person with the disorder may or may not be fully aware of the abnormality of the situation, but still takes effort to hide the disorder to other people. And because the scars run deep in one's emotions, it is easier to hide, because of the inner conflicts that the situation creates and brings out.

Harming one's self then becomes a cycle that is hard to stop, because it goes beyond the surface layers of the skin. It is symptomatic of psychological, physical, and emotional trauma that the skin picker may have experienced at some point in their life.

While obsessive-compulsive disorder is a means to protect the person from external factors that may cause him/her pain, skin picking is a person's attempt to guard his or herself from external pain, which they see as inevitable and expected.

With skin picking and self-harm, the person is able to be in control of causing just the right amount of pain. By inflicting pain on themselves, it somehow lessens the blow of pain caused by external factors. This is similar to when someone cuts themselves to distract him/her from external pain, by causing internal pain that they can control.

Some of these outside forces or factors that cause pain in a person and drives them to pick their skin may be genuine or embellished in his/her head. The trouble is, when the disorder involves wild imagination that triggers self-damage, this can be a sign of a chemical imbalance in the brain, which is also common in the diagnosis of depression, obsessive-compulsive disorder, and other conditions.

Both obsessive-compulsive disorder and compulsive skin picking spawn during times of emotional turmoil and stress. Both of these serve as ways to get out of problems or as a disturbing means to confront them.

Skin picking eventually disconnects people from reality, and over time, they begin to find the activity as natural and pleasurable, as normal everyday things that people do. It becomes "part of them" and really distorts what normal pain should feel like.

When a person picks their skin to a point where they are no longer thinking about the action in which they are involved in, it is apparent that it has begun to become a disorder. People in their immediate environment will find this strange and are usually the ones to stop them from relentlessly harming themselves.

More often than not, however, people with a compulsive skin picking disorder don't talk about it with other people. They will, in fact, do everything they can to deny the problem. This creates tension and conflict in their social life, because they are constantly feeling like they need to hide something and can't be their authentic selves around the people that they care about.

This is a sad truth that inhibits the medical community to discover more about the disorder. More researchers can pave the way to more possibilities of discoveries, like its connection with obsessive-compulsive disorder, and this can lead to new and better ways of treatment.

However, because of the nature of the disorder and how pickers feel about it, compulsive skin pickers will not be open with their ailments, and it has severely limited the advancement of research.

Eating Disorders

Skin picking is a symptom that is sometimes found in people with eating disorders. People that suffer from eating disorders sometimes use skin picking as a way to manage emotions, as they experience relief and pleasure in the process of picking their skin. It is also used as a distraction to a more serious problem that is causing their eating disorder.

Since skin picking has no direct medicinal treatment, people with eating disorders that compulsively pick their skin are treated with anti-depressants to regulate distress and anxiety in order to help them cope with depression.

This route doesn't usually help the picker long-term, however, because the anti-depressants are just a cover for the internal issue, and actually delay the process that the picker must go through psychologically.

Addiction

Skin picking is also sometimes associated with addiction to illegal substances. Pickers start with scratching on one location of the body, promising to stop, but ending up bruising the entire stretch of skin on the body, one more pimple, one more scab, until the digging never stops.

Some people have overcome their addiction with alcohol, cigarettes and illegal substances, but not skin picking. Some experts say that it is just as addictive, because even when they are not skin picking, they are thinking about skin picking. It seems they have found a way to suppress other feelings and replace them with the pleasure of scratching the skin.

To suppress pain, negative feelings and emotions, one needs the release of endorphins to give a high and to be spared from pain.

While substance addicts get their source of endorphins from their substances, people that have a compulsive skin picking disorder are bound to experience the same high and endorphin rush with skin picking.

According to many accounts, the pain does not come at once, but rather builds up in a trance. The pain and shame comes usually around thirty minutes later, as the inevitable pile of skin on the floor has to be picked up.

People with skin picking problems have also learned to be discreet about their condition, and they learn to be so in the harshest way possible. Upon realizing they have mutilated their bodies, they usually try their best to cover these bruises and avoid opportunities that might lead to questions about their condition.

Most of these people also have had experiences being caught with a bloody finger and had to grope for explanations, because they feel like it is simply impossible for other people to understand.

Unfortunately, there are more possibilities of healing for addiction than skin picking. People with this disorder do want to stop, but it is not as simple as taking a prescription drug from your doctor. Treatment for skin picking is fixed psychologically and takes a lot of mental strength from the person who is dealing with it.

Medication is usually directed to heal psychiatric conditions, so the person won't feel the need for self-relief, but if the person stops taking the medication, their skin picking will continue again. Therapy is geared towards practicing techniques to lessen anxiety and depression and to help people better manage their emotions. If combined, both medication and therapy can be helpful in healing.

Dermatophagia

Another common effect of skin picking is dermatophagia, or the compulsive disorder of a person who bites or eats his/her own skin. Usually this starts with biting around the nails, which could lead to discoloration and bleeding overtime.

While it is linked to skin picking, dermatophagia is considered to be an impulsive behavior that may be present with obsessive thoughts and anxiety. Apart from chewing skin around the nails, they could also do it on other parts of the body, which could then lead to more scabs or blisters - giving them another reason to hide their skin from others, for fear of scrutiny.

This behavior may then be bolstered by unpleasant events and times of apprehension in one's life. It could also be a never-ending cycle because when blisters are prevalent, one might be tempted to pull or bite them, which then might cause infection, even when one is not aware   of   it.

Chapter 5:

Overcoming Compulsive Skin Picking

Now that we understand what compulsive skin picking is, the causes of it, and the identity of those who suffer from it, it is time for us to look at some practical solutions. Let's cover specific ideas that have been proven to work for many people around the world, as well as the practical exercises that you can begin doing today!

Get rid of pins, tweezers, or even scissors - and anything else that you could use to mutilate the skin. If the need for them arises, you will be forced to borrow one from your friend or neighbor. The key here is to make sure that you do not surround yourself with "temptation" so that you won't undergo a relapse.

Avoid stressful situations with family and friends.

This first one may seem obvious, but it is one of the hardest for people to do. We spend most of our time around family and friends, and for many people, this is their picking stimulus. Just because someone is your family or friend, it doesn't mean they are beneficial to you.

You need to evaluate your friends and ask yourself, "Is this friendship helping me become a better person?" If the answer is no, this person may be causing stress in your life, and you may just be used to suppressing and dealing with it.

Even family can sometimes be unhealthy for you. Remember, if you are in a family situation that is not emotionally healthy, and you feel threatened or intimidated, this is most likely the cause of your skin picking. Unfortunately, it is very common for teenagers to pick their skin if they have a stressful relationship with one or both of their parents.

If you are unable to avoid the person you feel stressed around, make sure to tell that person that you are uncomfortable when they act a certain way. It would be best to show them the picking it has caused, but you may not be willing to show them your skin. It is ok if you do not feel comfortable with that. However, make sure to at least tell them that you would prefer them not to act that way around you, because it makes you feel uncomfortable. Remember, they may have no idea what you are going through, so don't hold back your feelings, because the only person you are hurting in the long run is yourself.

Switch activities when you feel a stressful stimulus.

When you notice yourself becoming stressed within a certain situation, maybe you have a test coming up at school or a deadline approaching at work, do your best to find something you can mess with other than your skin.

Good examples that have worked for people are using a stress ball that you can squeeze or chewing some gum. Sometimes, if you put 5 or 6 pieces of gum in your mouth, you can distract yourself from picking, because you will be preoccupied with the difficulty of chewing that much gum at once.

Wear full body clothing to prevent yourself from being able to pick.

Wearing a long-sleeve shirt and pants, as well as socks, can help prevent picking an area under your clothes. When you wake up in the morning, the first thing you should do is put on a full layer of clothing to cover the areas where you are most susceptible to pick.

Make sure you do this in the morning, so you are not allowing the possibility for you to start picking at your weak spots. It is much easier to stop picking at an area when it is completely covered than it is to stop picking at bare skin.

Remember that you may feel uncomfortable, at first, while doing this, because you will really want to pick at your favorite spots.

But remember, if you can get through the first few days, just think about how your skin will heal and the confidence you will have in the near future.

Depending on how serious you are and how far you are willing to go, you can even wear gloves to prevent yourself from picking at all. This will seem weird at first, but depending on how open you want to be with others, it can quickly speed up your recovery.

Meditation

You know why so many people are getting inclined to meditate? Well, for one, meditating helps you relax and also drives stress away. This way, especially if you meditate in the morning, you can be sure that you'll feel good for the rest of the day and so you will also be able to do what you have to do with much less emotional resistance. Meditation also improves heart rate and metabolism, mitigates insomnia, and normalizes blood pressure, amongst other benefits.

Mediation has been proven to help people who struggle with depression, anxiety and stress. Meditating for 20 minutes a day can make a world of difference for someone who feels the need to pick. When you meditate, you clear your mind completely, and it allows you to look at everything around you in a much more objective way.

You won't get as emotionally caught up in all the little stresses of your life, which will help you to pinpoint what you are getting stressed or worried about in the first place. Ideally, you can meditate in the morning because it will clear your mind for the upcoming day. Also, you'll be operating on much less momentum at the beginning of the day, so it will be easier to "make time" for.

Make sure to choose a quiet spot in your home where you can sit on the floor, or where you can place a cushion or a yoga mat to sit on. Some people also create their own altar, with candles and inspiring photos, but it's up to you if you want to do this as well. Just make sure that the space you choose is quiet and that no one will bother you.

Meditation is also about learning how to relax and breathe freely. Make sure that you loosen your face and neck, together with your stomach and hands, and that you breathe through the nose. Just focus on softening and relaxing all the parts of your body and let go of any tension that you might be holding.

Eating a whole foods based diet and foods that encourage endorphin production.

A whole foods based diet is basically a diet that our caveman ancestors would eat. It doesn't contain any processed foods, just meats, beans, veggies, fruits, and anything that naturally grows from the ground. This can be very helpful to a picker in multiple ways.

When your diet is filled with processed sugars and corn syrup, your brain doesn't function properly and can go into a "haze". This haze can sometimes prevent you from taking action on the important things in life and forces you to stay in your current situation, even if you have the desire to make a change for the better. It is important to have a clear mind when trying to overcome such an addicting habit as compulsive skin picking.

This type of diet will also give you clearer skin, because many forms of acne are caused by our current diets, due to the high concentration of sugars and chemicals that we do not digest well. Eating a cleaner diet will result in cleaner skin, which becomes a cycle from which you will benefit!

Eat foods that encourage endorphin production. As mentioned earlier, endorphins are the chemicals in your brain that make you feel happy. These are the same chemicals that are released when a person has an orgasm, completes an important task, and yes, even picks their skin.

Eating a diet rich in foods that encourage endorphin production will keep you in a better mood, which will help you when you feel vulnerable to start picking. Especially remember to eat the following foods when you know you may start feeling stressed soon.

Here is a list of 4 foods that encourage endorphin production: vanilla, ginseng, chocolate (small amounts), and peppers. Blueberries also help your brain to function at its best.

Exercise

One of the most effective ways to improve general well-being is exercise. First off, it improves skin conditions, which lessens the triggers for one to pick their skin. It improves one's appearance and attitude towards life, making you feel more positive. When one has exercised, he/she is also able to manage his/her emotions much better.

It only takes a few minutes a day to exercise, but the effects are invaluable. It keeps one focused and alert. There is no need to suppress negative feelings and the urge to self-mutilate.

When starting off, try exercising for a good seven minutes per day. Why 7? Research has it that seven minutes is good because it will not take much of your time, and yet it's sufficient to keep those "I want to go back to sleep" feelings at bay. Try brisk walking, or jogging, or do simple exercises such as Jumping Jacks, or a few squats, and you'll surely perk up.

Exercise also manages stress, which you may have otherwise taken out on yourself later that day. It even revives hormone levels, which helps keep the skin healthy and keep off excess weight. If you get into the habit of working out, you can tell yourself, whenever you feel like picking, you are going to take all of your stress out later that day on the weights at the gym or running at the park.

Avoid tight fitting clothing in the areas you like to pick.

One of the ways to indirectly stop skin picking is to stop the itchiness and irritation that is caused by common skin problems, such as acne.

To help eliminate another skin picking trigger, one should avoid clothes that are too tight and constrictive, because they can create a great deal of heat and friction between the skin and clothing.

Have a good, solid daily skin regimen and make sure to exfoliate.

Again, this may not directly stop the compulsive skin picking problem, but following healthy habits improve physical, emotional, and mental conditions. When you feel clean, you will look good and feel good.

These feelings are able to ignite a positive vibe that can help manage worries and anxieties. Taking care of the skin can be as simple as washing one's face regularly or scrubbing in the shower.

In the process of trying to stop skin picking, one should learn how to keep the skin clear and clean in order to avoid triggers. Make exfoliating a part of your daily skin regimen to ensure that the pores are not clogged, and those dead skin cells are removed in the shower in order to make way for new, healthy ones. You will feel cleaner, and your skin will be less irritated each day you continue to do this.

In order to get on a good skin regimen, it would be helpful to know whether your skin is dry, oily, or a combination of both. This information can be given to you by a dermatologist. It's also best to check if you have sensitive skin, as to avoid using products that may damage your skin all the more. A rule of thumb here is to use something natural and gentle in order to give the skin the kind of care that it needs.

Also, make sure to put on sunscreen. This is so you can protect yourself from the debilitating effects of the sun. Use those with at least SPF30. Re-apply sunscreen at least every 2 hours if spending extended time in sunlight.

It's also really important to moisturize in order to keep your skin from drying out and to seal in moisture that's important to keep the skin healthy. By giving your skin time, you won't be tempted to do your old habits again and let them rule your life. Just remember to take care of the skin daily - regularly - and not just when you feel like it.

Get enough sleep to think clearly.

This goes along with your diet. Not sleeping enough can cause major problems in your thinking. The last thing you want during the day is to become so tired that you aren't able to mentally keep yourself from picking at your skin again.

It is so frustrating to stop picking for a few days, and then start again because you didn't get enough sleep the night before, which lowers your defenses and makes you mentally lazy.

Sleeping also gives the body an opportunity to repair. For people with a history of skin picking, skin repair during sleep is vital. Try to get at least seven to eight hours of sleep each night.

Sleep is the best answer to stress, anxieties, and other negative emotions. With proper sleep, one is able to manage different emotions with focus and presence of mind. Don't underestimate this one!

Stimulus Control Training & Habit Reversal Training (HBT)

You can also undergo Stimulus Control Training, where you'd be able to alter your physical environment so you'd have less chances of picking the skin. As an example, if you're fond of picking the face, you may put some band-aids or tape on your face so you wouldn't be tempted to use your hands there.

You can also try Habit Reversal Training (HBT). This is a Cognitive Behavioral Treatment that allows you to identify the triggers of your skin picking. Your therapist would then teach you how you could cope with each given situation, especially when they arise and you feel like you have no control in the situation. The goal is to know how to manage your harmful urges before they take over your body.

For example, you'd be told to just clutch or scratch a stuffed toy, or use a finger toy in order to stop yourself from picking the skin. Finding other hobbies such as knitting, crocheting, or cross-stitching may also be helpful, but you may also need supervision so you would not be tempted to use the needles or pins on yourself. Ask your doctor about this.

Keeping your family, friends, or support network in the loop.

It was mentioned earlier that you don't NEED to tell your family and friends about your skin picking if you are not comfortable. However, your goal should be to ultimately tell the people who care about you sooner rather than later.

The reason this is so important, is that it creates some type of accountability for you to overcome the problem, as well as a small support system, even if it is just one person who knows about your struggle.

No matter what we are trying to accomplish in life, if we are accountable to somebody else, it will always help us accomplish that goal quicker, because we can't just back out whenever we want.

It is important to understand that no matter how bad of a situation your skin is in, you are better off telling the people close to you, because they are not going to care how bad it is; they want you to be happy.

Since the family comprises a person's immediate environment, it is only wise to make them a part of the treatment process. People with this disorder usually clam up because of the judgment they get from the people around them. Although these reactions are sometimes valid, they inevitably trigger further picking.

If you can, find a group in your city or town with people who suffer from compulsive skin picking as well. If there is no local group, look online for forums. There are many forums dedicated to people in the exact same situation as you.

The best part about these online forums is that you do not need to show your face or body, yet you can still share your struggles and triumphs, and receive very insightful tips that can help you on your way.

Conclusion

Hopefully this short, concise book was able to provide you with some practical, useful information. These are the strategies and information that has worked for people in the past and will continue to work in the future. If you stay consistent, they will work for you as well. Be optimistic about your current situation and make small progress each day!

This guide was meant to get you to understand the major factors and strategies regarding skin picking, but if you want to continue your research in a more extended manner, simply delve further into the topics that were discussed here.

Thank you and good luck in your own journey! You are not alone!